BALANCED BLISS: A COMPREHENSIVE GUIDE TO A HEALTHIER YOU

For further information:

doveland6@gmail.com

International standard book No:

SBN: 9798874015152

TABLE OF CONTENTS

INTRODUCTION

Welcome to "The Holistic Wellness Journey: A Comprehensive Guide to Health and Happiness." In the fast-paced and ever-evolving landscape of health and wellness, this book serves as your compass, offering a comprehensive and practical guide to empower you on a transformative journey towards holistic well-being. As we navigate the pages of this book, we embark on a profound exploration of the intricate connections between nutrition, exercise, mindfulness, and the mind-body connection, all converging to shape a life of sustained health, happiness, and fulfillment.

The Holistic Wellness Philosophy: At the heart of this book lies a holistic wellness philosophy that transcends the narrow confines of fad diets and quick fixes. Holistic wellness encapsulates a multidimensional approach, recognizing that true well-being extends beyond physical health to encompass mental, emotional, and even spiritual dimensions. Our journey is not just about achieving a number on the scale; it's about fostering a harmonious and balanced existence where every facet of your being thrives.

The Structure of the Book: "The Holistic Wellness Journey" unfolds across 15 enriching chapters, each meticulously crafted to guide you through distinct aspects of holistic health. From understanding the fundamentals of nutrition and exercise to cultivating a positive mind-body connection, the chapters form a cohesive narrative, building upon one another to provide a comprehensive roadmap for your well-being.

• **Foundational Knowledge**: Begin your journey by establishing a solid foundation in nutrition with chapters 1 to 4. Explore the significance of mindful eating, the role of macronutrients, and the impact of diet on energy levels.

• **Mindful Living**: Delve into the world of mindfulness and conscious living in chapters 5 to 9. Discover the transformative power of mindful eating, stress management, and positive thinking as you cultivate a more profound connection between your mind and body.

• **Navigating Challenges**: Chapters 10 to 12 equip you with strategies to navigate social situations, overcome obstacles, and stay on track. Learn how to make healthy choices in various scenarios and build resilience for the inevitable challenges on your wellness journey.

• **Exercise and Nutrition Synergy**: In Chapter 11, explore the dynamic relationship between exercise and nutrition, uncovering how these elements synergize to optimize your fitness outcomes.

• **Long-Term Wellness**: As we approach the conclusion of our journey, Chapters 13 to 15 provide insights into sustainable weight management, the mind-body connection, and setting future wellness goals. Embrace a holistic approach to well-being that extends beyond short-term fixes to create lasting and meaningful changes.

Your Empowerment Toolkit: Embedded within each chapter are practical tools, actionable insights, and engaging exercises designed to empower you on your wellness journey. From mindful eating practices and stress-management techniques to personalized goal-setting exercises, this book is more than a guide—it's a hands-on toolkit for transformative change.

Embark on Your Journey: Whether you're at the beginning of your wellness expedition or seeking to deepen your understanding, "The Holistic Wellness Journey" invites you to embark on a transformative exploration. This book is not a one-size-fits-all prescription but a personalized guide, encouraging you to embrace a sustainable and holistic approach to health and happiness.

Get ready to embark on a journey that transcends the limitations of temporary fixes, embraces the richness of holistic wellness, and empowers you to live a life of sustained health and happiness. Your journey starts now.

DEDICATION

To all those who embark on the transformative journey of holistic wellness,

This book is dedicated to you—the seekers, the dreamers, the resilient souls committed to nurturing your health and happiness. In the pages that follow, may you find inspiration, guidance, and the tools to create a life of sustained well-being.

To the tireless explorers of mindful living, balanced nutrition, and the intricate dance between body and mind, this dedication is a tribute to you. Your commitment to holistic health is a beacon, lighting the way for others to follow.

May your journey be filled with self-discovery, resilience in the face of challenges, and the joy that comes from cultivating a harmonious existence. Here's to a life lived with intention, where each choice is a step towards health, happiness, and the fulfillment of your unique wellness journey.

With gratitude and best wishes for your holistic well-being,

Justin Hunt.

Chapter one

UNDERSTANDING NUTRITIONAL BASICS

The journey to a healthier lifestyle begins with a solid understanding of nutritional basics. In this foundational chapter, we delve into the essential components of a balanced diet and the key principles that underpin optimal nutrition.

Macronutrients and Micronutrients:

•	Macronutrients, including carbohydrates, proteins, and fats, are the building blocks of our diet. Understanding their roles and incorporating them in appropriate proportions is crucial for overall health.

•	Micronutrients, such as vitamins and minerals, play vital roles in various physiological processes. We explore the importance of these micronutrients and their food sources.

Importance of a Balanced Diet:

•	A balanced diet is not about deprivation but about nourishing your body with the right nutrients in the right amounts.

•	We discuss the impact of a balanced diet on energy levels, metabolism, and overall well-being.

•	Highlighting the relationship between nutrition and chronic diseases, we emphasize the preventive aspects of maintaining a balanced lifestyle.

Dietary Guidelines and Recommendations:

• We explore established dietary guidelines and recommendations from reputable health organizations.

• Breaking down these guidelines into practical tips, readers will gain insights into creating meals that align with their nutritional needs.

Personalized Nutrition:

• Every individual is unique, and one-size-fits-all approaches may not be effective. This section guides readers on personalizing their nutrition plans based on factors like age, gender, activity level, and health status.

• Understanding dietary preferences and cultural considerations, we encourage readers to create sustainable and enjoyable eating habits.

Holistic Approach to Nutrition:

• Nutrition is not just about what you eat; it's also about how you eat. We introduce the concept of mindful eating and the importance of savoring each bite.

• The chapter emphasizes the interconnectedness of nutrition with other aspects of life, such as sleep, stress management, and mental well-being.

By the end of Chapter 1, readers will have a solid grasp of the fundamental principles of nutrition, setting the stage for the practical application of this knowledge throughout the book. Armed with this understanding, they will be better equipped to make informed choices that align with their health and wellness goals.

Chapter Two

SETTING REALISTIC GOALS

Embarking on a journey towards a healthier lifestyle requires clear objectives and a roadmap for success. Chapter 2 focuses on the importance of setting realistic and achievable goals, guiding readers through the process of establishing a foundation for effective and sustainable change.

Understanding the Significance of Goals:

•	Goals provide direction, motivation, and a sense of purpose in the pursuit of a healthier lifestyle.

•	We discuss the psychological and physiological benefits of goal-setting, emphasizing how it contributes to long-term success.

SMART Goals:

•	Introducing the SMART criteria (Specific, Measurable, Achievable, Relevant, Time-Bound), we guide readers in creating goals that are clear, tangible, and attainable.

•	Providing examples and exercises, readers learn to transform vague aspirations into concrete, actionable steps.

Short-Term vs. Long-Term Goals:

- Distinguishing between short-term and long-term goals, we explore their respective roles in the overall journey.

- Short-term goals create stepping stones, fostering a sense of accomplishment, while long-term goals offer a broader vision and purpose.

Tailoring Goals to Individual Needs:

- Recognizing that everyone's journey is unique, we guide readers in tailoring goals to their personal preferences, lifestyle, and health status.

- Encouraging flexibility, we emphasize the importance of adapting goals as circumstances evolve.

Breaking Down Goals into Actionable Steps:

- Breaking down larger goals into smaller, manageable tasks enhances clarity and feasibility.

- Readers are provided with strategies to create a step-by-step plan, making the pursuit of their goals more achievable.

Overcoming Challenges and Obstacles:

• Anticipating and addressing potential challenges is integral to goal achievement. We discuss common obstacles and provide practical solutions to overcome them.

• Emphasizing resilience, readers are empowered to navigate setbacks and stay committed to their objectives.

Celebrating Milestones:

• Acknowledging progress, no matter how small, is crucial for maintaining motivation. We discuss the importance of celebrating achievements and setting new milestones.

Periodic Goal Review:

• Regularly reviewing and reassessing goals allows for adjustments and ensures continued progress.

• We provide guidance on assessing achievements, modifying goals, and staying motivated for the long haul.

By the end of Chapter 2, readers will have developed a clear understanding of the role goals play in their journey to a healthier lifestyle. Armed with SMART objectives, tailored to their unique circumstances, they will be equipped with the tools to navigate challenges and celebrate successes along the way.

Chapter Three

BUILDING A STRONG FOUNDATION

Building a strong nutritional foundation is paramount in achieving and maintaining a healthy lifestyle. Chapter 3 delves into the crucial aspects of selecting the right foods and understanding the role of various food groups in promoting overall well-being.

The Importance of Whole Foods:

• Whole foods are minimally processed and retain their natural nutrients. We explore the benefits of incorporating whole grains, fruits, vegetables, lean proteins, and healthy fats into the diet.

• Highlighting the connection between whole foods and enhanced nutrient absorption, readers gain insight into the impact on energy levels and vitality.

Understanding Macronutrients:

•   A detailed examination of macronutrients—carbohydrates, proteins, and fats—provides readers with a foundational understanding of their roles in the body.

•   We emphasize the importance of balance, dispelling common misconceptions about certain macronutrients.

Choosing the Right Carbohydrates:

•   Carbohydrates are a primary source of energy. The chapter guides readers in selecting complex carbohydrates, such as whole grains and vegetables, while moderating refined sugars.

•   Practical tips for managing carbohydrate intake are provided, considering individual needs and preferences.

Embracing Lean Proteins:

•   Proteins are essential for muscle repair and overall body function. We explore various lean protein sources, including plant-based options, and address concerns related to protein intake.

• Recipes and meal ideas featuring lean proteins cater to diverse dietary preferences.

Incorporating Healthy Fats:

• Healthy fats are crucial for brain health, hormone production, and nutrient absorption. We discuss sources of monounsaturated and polyunsaturated fats and their role in a balanced diet.

• Practical guidance on cooking with healthy fats and making mindful choices is included.

Micronutrients and Antioxidants:

• Micronutrients, such as vitamins and minerals, play a vital role in supporting various physiological functions. We highlight the importance of consuming a diverse range of nutrient-rich foods.

• Antioxidants, found in fruits and vegetables, are explored for their role in combating oxidative stress and promoting longevity.

Hydration and Its Impact:

• The significance of proper hydration is discussed, emphasizing its role in digestion, metabolism, and overall well-being.

• Creative ways to stay hydrated, including infused water recipes, are provided to make this essential habit enjoyable.

Practical Application:

• Readers are guided on translating theoretical knowledge into practical application. Sample meal plans and recipes are included, showcasing the integration of whole, nutrient-dense foods into everyday life.

By the end of Chapter 3, readers will have gained a comprehensive understanding of building a strong nutritional foundation. Armed with knowledge about whole foods, macronutrients, and micronutrients, they will be better equipped to make informed choices that support their health and wellness goals.

Chapter Four

MASTERING PORTION CONTROL

Portion control is a crucial aspect of maintaining a balanced diet and achieving sustainable weight management. In this chapter, we explore the principles and practices of mastering portion control, providing readers with tools to make mindful and healthful choices when it comes to serving sizes.

The Importance of Portion Control:

•	Portion control is key to preventing overeating and maintaining a healthy weight.

•	Understanding the difference between portion size and serving size sets the stage for making informed decisions about food consumption.

Visualizing Portion Sizes:

•	Visual cues are powerful tools for estimating portion sizes without relying on measuring tools.

•	The chapter provides practical visuals and comparisons, empowering readers to gauge appropriate portions at a glance.

Using Everyday Objects as Portion Guides:

•	Everyday items, such as your hand, can serve as convenient guides for portion control.

•	Readers are introduced to various household objects that can assist in estimating appropriate portions for different food groups.

The Plate Method:

• The plate method involves dividing a meal visually to ensure a balanced intake of macronutrients.

• We discuss the plate method in detail, offering insights into how it promotes a balanced diet and supports weight management.

Mindful Eating Techniques:

• Mindful eating involves being present and attentive during meals, fostering a better connection with hunger and fullness cues.

• Practical techniques, such as savoring each bite, chewing mindfully, and recognizing satiety, are explored.

Strategies for Eating Out:

• Dining out can present challenges in portion control. We provide tips for navigating restaurant menus, controlling portions, and making healthier choices.

• Techniques for managing social situations and peer pressure are also discussed.

Importance of Reading Food Labels:

• Reading food labels is crucial for understanding portion sizes, nutritional content, and making informed choices.

• We guide readers on deciphering food labels, focusing on key elements that impact portion control.

Portion Control for Snacking:

• Snacking can be a pitfall for overeating. The chapter addresses healthy snacking habits and provides examples of portion-controlled snacks.

• Readers learn how to incorporate snacks into their day without compromising their overall nutritional goals.

Adapting Portion Control to Individual Needs:

• Recognizing that individual needs vary, we discuss tailoring portion control to factors like age, activity level, and weight loss or maintenance goals.

• Encouraging flexibility, readers are empowered to make adjustments based on their unique circumstances.

Monitoring Progress:

• Regularly monitoring portion control habits is essential for long-term success.

• We provide tools and techniques for tracking progress, making adjustments, and celebrating achievements in mastering portion control.

By the end of Chapter 4, readers will have a comprehensive understanding of mastering portion control as a fundamental skill in achieving and maintaining a healthy lifestyle. Armed with practical techniques and strategies, they will be well-equipped to make mindful choices about their food intake, supporting their overall wellness goals.

Chapter Five

THE POWER OF HYDRATION

Hydration is a fundamental aspect of overall well-being, influencing various physiological functions. Chapter 5 explores the importance of staying adequately hydrated and provides practical insights into maintaining optimal fluid balance for enhanced health.

Understanding the Role of Hydration:

•   Water is essential for life, comprising a significant portion of the human body and playing a vital role in various bodily functions.

•   This section delves into the physiological importance of hydration, including temperature regulation, digestion, nutrient transport, and toxin elimination.

Daily Hydration Needs:

•   Individual hydration needs vary based on factors such as age, gender, activity level, and climate.

•   We provide guidelines for estimating daily water intake requirements, empowering readers to tailor their hydration goals to personal circumstances.

Signs of Dehydration:

•	Recognizing the signs of dehydration is crucial for prompt intervention. We discuss common indicators, such as dark urine, thirst, and fatigue, emphasizing the importance of staying vigilant.

Creative Hydration Strategies:

•	Drinking enough water doesn't have to be mundane. This section offers creative and enjoyable ways to stay hydrated, including infused water recipes, herbal teas, and hydrating foods.

•	Emphasizing the variety of sources contributing to hydration, readers discover alternatives beyond plain water.

Balancing Fluid Intake:

•	Achieving a balance between water and other beverages contributes to overall hydration. We explore the impact of various drinks, including tea, coffee, and milk, on fluid balance.

- Practical tips for moderating the consumption of sugary and caffeinated beverages are provided.

Hydration and Exercise:

- Physical activity increases the body's demand for fluids. This section addresses the importance of hydrating before, during, and after exercise, tailoring recommendations to different types and intensities of physical activity.

- Electrolyte balance and the role of sports drinks are discussed in the context of exercise-related hydration needs.

Hydration Challenges and Solutions:

- Overcoming common hydration challenges, such as forgetfulness and dislike of plain water, is essential. Practical solutions, including hydration reminders, reusable water bottles, and flavor infusions, are explored.

- Strategies for maintaining hydration during travel and busy schedules are also discussed.

Water Quality and Safety:

• Ensuring the quality and safety of water sources is paramount. We provide guidance on selecting clean and safe drinking water, including tips for filtering and purifying water when necessary.

Special Considerations:

• Individuals with specific health conditions, such as pregnant women and older adults, may have unique hydration needs. This section addresses special considerations for these populations.

• We also discuss hydration during illness and recovery, emphasizing the importance of adapting fluid intake based on individual circumstances.

Hydration as a Lifestyle:

• Cultivating a habit of staying hydrated is a lifestyle choice. We discuss the psychological and behavioral aspects of making hydration a consistent and integral part of daily life.

• Readers are encouraged to view hydration as a proactive and empowering step towards better health.

By the end of Chapter 5, readers will have gained a comprehensive understanding of the power of hydration and its profound impact on overall well-being. Armed with practical strategies and insights, they will be well-equipped to make informed choices to maintain optimal fluid balance and support their health and vitality.

Chapter Six

SUPER FOODS FOR SUPER YOU

Super foods, nutrient-dense foods packed with health benefits, play a pivotal role in supporting overall well-being. Chapter 6 explores the concept of super foods, their nutritional profiles, and provides practical ways to incorporate these powerhouse ingredients into a balanced diet.

Defining Super foods:

• Superfoods are natural, whole foods that are rich in essential nutrients, antioxidants, and other beneficial compounds.

• We discuss the criteria that classify foods as superfoods and address common misconceptions surrounding this term.

Nutrient-Rich Powerhouses:

• Superfoods are often high in vitamins, minerals, antioxidants, and phytochemicals. This section explores the nutritional content of popular superfoods, such as berries, leafy greens, nuts, seeds, and fatty fish.

• Emphasizing variety, readers learn about the diverse range of nutrients available from different superfoods.

Benefits of Superfoods:

•	The chapter details the specific health benefits associated with consuming superfoods, including improved heart health, enhanced immune function, and potential disease prevention.

•	Scientific evidence supporting the positive impact of superfoods on various aspects of health is presented.

Incorporating Superfoods into the Diet:

•	Practical tips and creative recipes are provided to help readers seamlessly integrate superfoods into their meals and snacks.

•	Sample meal plans showcase balanced and flavorful combinations featuring a variety of superfoods.

Everyday Superfoods:

•	Many superfoods are readily available and can be part of daily dietary habits. This section introduces readers to common superfoods that are easily accessible, emphasizing simplicity and convenience.

•	The chapter explores how everyday superfoods can be used in diverse culinary applications.

Seasonal Superfoods:

• Superfoods can vary by season, offering an opportunity to diversify one's diet throughout the year. We discuss seasonal superfoods, their nutritional benefits, and ways to incorporate them into seasonal menus.

Plant-Based Superfoods:

• Plant-based superfoods, such as quinoa, chia seeds, and kale, are rich in nutrients and contribute to a sustainable and environmentally friendly diet.

• Readers discover the benefits of incorporating more plant-based superfoods and receive guidance on plant-based meal planning.

Superfood Supplements:

• While whole foods are ideal, some may consider supplements for added convenience. We discuss the pros and cons of superfood supplements and provide guidelines for choosing high-quality options.

Balanced Superfood Consumption:

• Moderation and variety are key when incorporating superfoods. The chapter discusses the importance of a well-rounded diet and how superfoods can complement other nutrient sources.

•	Readers are encouraged to view superfoods as part of a holistic approach to nutrition.

Culinary Creativity with Superfoods:

•	Superfoods can be delicious and versatile ingredients in the kitchen. We provide cooking tips, flavor pairings, and culinary techniques to enhance the enjoyment of superfoods in everyday meals.

By the end of Chapter 6, readers will have a comprehensive understanding of superfoods and their potential impact on health. Armed with practical strategies for incorporating these nutrient-rich foods into their diets, readers can make informed choices that contribute to overall well-being and vitality.

Chapter Seven

MEAL PLANNING MADE EASY

Effective meal planning is a cornerstone of a healthy and sustainable dietary lifestyle. Chapter 7 delves into the art and science of meal planning, offering readers practical tools, strategies, and inspiration to streamline their approach to nutrition.

The Importance of Meal Planning:

•	Meal planning is a proactive strategy that helps individuals make intentional and nutritious food choices.

•	We discuss how meal planning contributes to better time management, reduced stress, and improved adherence to nutritional goals.

Tailoring Meal Plans to Individual Needs:

•	Recognizing that one-size-fits-all meal plans may not be practical, the chapter guides readers in customizing their meal plans based on factors such as dietary preferences, health goals, and lifestyle.

•	Tips for accommodating special dietary needs, such as vegetarianism or food allergies, are also included.

Components of a Balanced Meal:

•	A balanced meal incorporates a variety of macronutrients and micronutrients. We break down the essential components of a balanced plate and discuss portion sizes.

•	Practical examples and templates assist readers in creating well-rounded meals that support their nutritional needs.

Batch Cooking and Prep:

•	Batch cooking is a time-saving technique that involves preparing larger quantities of food to have on hand for future meals.

•	We provide step-by-step guidance on batch cooking and offer ideas for versatile ingredients that can be used in multiple dishes.

Efficient Grocery Shopping:

•   Strategic grocery shopping is a key element of successful meal planning. The chapter explores tips for creating a shopping list, navigating the grocery store, and making cost-effective choices.

•   Guidance on reading food labels and selecting fresh, seasonal produce is also provided.

Sunday Meal Prep Routine:

•   Establishing a weekly meal prep routine, such as a Sunday prep session, can streamline the cooking process and set the tone for a successful week.

•   We offer a sample meal prep routine and discuss how to adapt it to individual preferences and schedules.

Creating a Varied and Enjoyable Menu:

•   Variety is essential for maintaining interest and ensuring a diverse intake of nutrients. Readers learn how to create menus that are both nutritionally balanced and enjoyable.

•   The chapter includes tips for incorporating new recipes, exploring different cuisines, and experimenting with flavors.

Time-Saving Cooking Techniques:

•	Time-efficient cooking techniques, such as one-pot meals, sheet pan dinners, and slow cooking, are explored.

•	Readers discover how to maximize efficiency in the kitchen without compromising on the nutritional quality of their meals.

Adapting Meal Plans for Busy Schedules:

•	Busy schedules can pose challenges to meal planning. We discuss strategies for adapting meal plans to accommodate hectic days, including quick and easy recipes and portable meal options.

•	Readers are empowered to prioritize nutrition even in the midst of a busy lifestyle.

Mindful Eating Practices:

•	Mindful eating is an integral part of meal planning. The chapter introduces readers to the concept of mindful eating and provides tips for savoring meals, paying attention to hunger and fullness cues, and cultivating a positive relationship with food.

By the end of Chapter 7, readers will have acquired practical skills to simplify and enhance their meal planning process. Armed with the tools to create balanced, enjoyable, and convenient meals, they can make sustained progress towards their nutritional goals while adapting to the demands of their unique lifestyles.

Chapter Eight

EATING FOR ENERGY

Optimal energy levels are vital for overall well-being and productivity. Chapter 8 explores the connection between nutrition and sustained energy, providing readers with insights into the types of foods that support vitality and practical strategies for maintaining consistent energy levels throughout the day.

The Role of Macronutrients in Energy:

• Macronutrients, including carbohydrates, proteins, and fats, are the primary sources of energy for the body.

• This section delves into how each macronutrient contributes to energy production and the importance of a balanced intake for sustained vitality.

Complex Carbohydrates and Stable Blood Sugar:

• Complex carbohydrates, found in whole grains, fruits, and vegetables, provide a steady release of glucose, promoting stable blood sugar levels.

• Practical tips for incorporating complex carbohydrates into meals are discussed to support sustained energy.

Protein for Muscle Maintenance and Repair:

•   Protein plays a crucial role in muscle maintenance, repair, and overall body function.

•   We explore the importance of including adequate protein sources in the diet and offer examples of protein-rich foods for sustained energy.

Healthy Fats for Sustained Energy:

•   Healthy fats, such as those found in avocados, nuts, and olive oil, contribute to sustained energy by providing a concentrated source of calories and supporting nutrient absorption.

•   Strategies for incorporating healthy fats into meals and snacks are highlighted.

Balancing Macronutrients for Energy Stability:

•   Achieving a balance of macronutrients in each meal supports energy stability and prevents energy crashes.

•   Readers learn practical approaches to create well-balanced meals that provide sustained fuel for daily activities.

The Importance of Hydration for Energy:

•   Dehydration can lead to fatigue and decreased cognitive function. This section emphasizes the role of proper hydration in maintaining energy levels.

•   Readers are encouraged to establish hydration habits that complement their overall energy strategy.

Energy-Boosting Nutrients:

•   Certain vitamins and minerals, such as B-vitamins and iron, play a key role in energy metabolism.

•   We explore foods rich in these nutrients and how to incorporate them into a balanced diet for optimal energy production.

Timing of Meals and Snacks:

•   The timing of meals and snacks influences energy levels throughout the day. We discuss the importance of regular eating intervals and provide guidelines for incorporating energy-boosting snacks.

•   Tips for managing hunger and preventing energy dips between meals are included.

Pre-Workout and Post-Workout Nutrition:

• Fueling the body before and after exercise is essential for sustained energy and optimal recovery.

• This section offers recommendations for pre-workout and post-workout nutrition, addressing the unique energy needs associated with physical activity.

Mindful Eating for Energy:

• Mindful eating practices contribute to better digestion and nutrient absorption, enhancing overall energy levels.

• Readers are introduced to mindful eating techniques, such as eating without distractions and savoring each bite, to cultivate a positive relationship with food and support energy balance.

By the end of Chapter 8, readers will have gained a comprehensive understanding of how nutrition influences energy levels. Armed with practical strategies for incorporating energy-boosting foods into their diets and adopting mindful eating practices, they can take proactive steps towards sustaining vitality throughout their daily lives.

Chapter Nine

MINDFUL EATING

Mindful eating is a practice that fosters a deeper connection between individuals and their food, promoting a more conscious and enjoyable relationship with eating. Chapter 9 explores the principles and benefits of mindful eating, providing readers with practical techniques to enhance their overall well-being and relationship with food.

Understanding Mindful Eating:

•	Mindful eating involves being fully present and engaged in the eating experience, paying attention to the flavors, textures, and sensations of each bite.

• We discuss the contrast between mindful eating and mindless or distracted eating habits, highlighting the potential impact on overall health.

The Mind-Body Connection:

• Mindful eating is rooted in the mind-body connection, acknowledging the interplay between physical and emotional cues related to hunger and satiety.

• Readers gain insights into how mindfulness can influence eating behaviors and contribute to a more balanced approach to nourishment.

Cultivating Awareness of Hunger and Fullness:

• Mindful eating encourages individuals to recognize and respond to genuine hunger and fullness cues, fostering a more intuitive approach to eating.

• Practical exercises guide readers in developing awareness of their own hunger and fullness signals.

Slowing Down the Eating Process:

•	Eating slowly allows individuals to savor and appreciate each bite, aiding in digestion and promoting a sense of satisfaction.

•	Strategies for slowing down the eating process, including mindful chewing and setting utensils down between bites, are discussed.

Eliminating Distractions:

•	Mindful eating encourages the elimination of distractions during meals, such as electronic devices or work-related tasks.

•	We provide tips for creating a mindful eating environment, allowing individuals to focus on the sensory experience of their meals.

Savoring the Flavors:

•	Savoring the flavors of food enhances the enjoyment of meals and contributes to a more positive relationship with eating.

•	The chapter explores techniques for enhancing flavor awareness and savoring the diverse tastes in a variety of foods.

Emotional Eating and Mindful Awareness:

• Mindful eating addresses emotional eating by encouraging individuals to explore the emotional triggers behind their food choices.

• Practical approaches for navigating emotional eating and developing alternative coping mechanisms are discussed.

Overcoming Guilt and Judgment:

• Mindful eating promotes a non-judgmental attitude towards food choices, helping individuals overcome guilt or shame associated with eating.

• Readers learn techniques for developing a compassionate and accepting mindset toward their eating habits.

Mindful Eating in Social Settings:

• Eating mindfully can be practiced in social settings without sacrificing the joy of shared meals.

• We provide guidance on incorporating mindfulness into social gatherings and handling potential challenges with grace.

Making Mindful Eating a Daily Practice:

• Mindful eating is most effective when it becomes a daily practice. Readers are encouraged to integrate mindfulness into their eating routines gradually.

• We discuss practical tips for making mindful eating a sustainable and enjoyable part of everyday life.

By the end of Chapter 9, readers will have a thorough understanding of mindful eating principles and the potential positive impact on their relationship with food. Equipped with practical techniques, they can embark on a journey toward more conscious and fulfilling eating experiences, fostering a healthier and more balanced approach to nutrition.

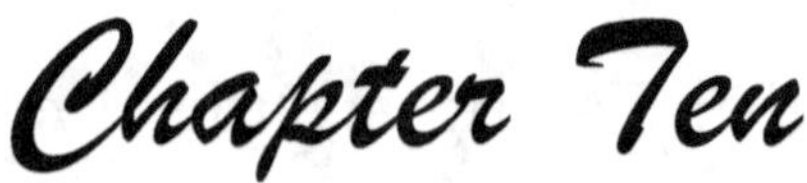

Chapter Ten

NAVIGATING SOCIAL SITUATIONS

Maintaining a healthy and balanced diet can sometimes be challenging in social settings, where external influences and peer pressure may come into play. Chapter 10 addresses the strategies and mindset needed to navigate various social situations without compromising one's nutritional goals.

Social Challenges to Healthy Eating:

• Social gatherings, parties, and events often present challenges to maintaining a balanced diet.

• This section explores common obstacles, such as the abundance of tempting but unhealthy food choices, and addresses the impact of social pressure on eating habits.

Strategies for Making Healthy Choices:

• Practical strategies are provided to empower individuals to make healthy food choices in social settings.

• Readers learn techniques for scanning menus, identifying healthier options, and creating a plan before attending events to stay on track.

Communicating Dietary Preferences:

• Open communication about dietary preferences and restrictions is essential. The chapter offers guidance on how to effectively communicate with hosts, friends, or colleagues about specific dietary needs.

• Tips for asserting one's choices without feeling awkward or isolated in social situations are discussed.

Bringing Healthy Options to Potlucks and Parties:

• Taking proactive steps to contribute healthy dishes to potlucks and parties ensures there are nutritious options available.

• We provide recipe ideas and tips for preparing shareable, wholesome dishes that everyone can enjoy.

Alcohol and Nutrition:

• Alcohol consumption can impact nutritional choices and overall health. This section discusses the potential effects of alcohol on food choices and provides guidelines for mindful drinking.

• Strategies for choosing lower-calorie and lower-sugar alcoholic beverages are included.

Handling Peer Pressure:

•	Peer pressure can be a significant factor in deviating from a healthy eating plan. Readers gain insights into recognizing and handling peer pressure gracefully.

•	Strategies for staying true to one's nutritional goals while still enjoying social interactions are explored.

Smart Eating at Restaurants:

•	Dining out is a common social activity that may pose challenges to healthy eating. The chapter provides practical tips for making smart choices at restaurants, including navigating menus and portion sizes.

•	Techniques for modifying orders to suit dietary preferences without feeling self-conscious are discussed.

Balancing Indulgences:

•	Enjoying occasional treats and indulgences is part of a balanced approach to nutrition. The chapter explores the concept of balance, providing guidance on how to enjoy special occasions without guilt.

• Tips for preventing overindulgence and bouncing back after occasional indulgences are included.

Mindful Eating in Social Settings:

• Mindful eating practices are particularly valuable in social settings. Readers are encouraged to apply mindful eating principles when faced with tempting or indulgent foods during social occasions.

• Techniques for savoring each bite and staying attuned to hunger and fullness cues are emphasized.

Cultivating a Positive Social Food Environment: - The chapter concludes by discussing the importance of cultivating a positive and supportive social food environment. - Strategies for influencing social circles positively, encouraging healthier choices, and fostering a collective commitment to well-being are explored.

By the end of Chapter 10, readers will have gained practical insights and strategies for navigating social situations while maintaining a balanced and healthy approach to eating. Armed with these tools, they can confidently participate in social events without compromising their nutritional goals, fostering a positive relationship with food in various social settings.

Chapter Eleven

EXERCISE AND NUTRITION SYNERGY

The relationship between exercise and nutrition is integral to achieving overall health and wellness. Chapter 11 explores how these two elements work synergistically, providing readers with insights into the role of nutrition in supporting physical activity and optimizing fitness outcomes.

Understanding the Interplay between Exercise and Nutrition:

•	Exercise and nutrition are interconnected components of a healthy lifestyle, each influencing the effectiveness of the other.

•	This section establishes the foundation for understanding how nutrition impacts energy levels, recovery, and performance during exercise.

The Importance of Proper Nutrition for Exercise:

•	Proper nutrition is essential for fueling the body before, during, and after exercise.

•	We discuss how adequate nutrient intake supports energy needs, enhances performance, and aids in recovery.

Pre-Exercise Nutrition:

•	The chapter explores the significance of pre-exercise nutrition in providing the necessary energy for physical activity.

•	Practical tips for choosing the right pre-exercise meals and snacks based on the type and intensity of the workout are provided.

Hydration and Exercise Performance:

- Proper hydration is crucial for optimal exercise performance and recovery.

- We delve into the impact of dehydration on physical performance and offer guidelines for maintaining adequate fluid balance before, during, and after exercise.

Nutrition during Exercise:

- For prolonged or intense physical activity, nutritional support during exercise becomes important.

- Strategies for consuming appropriate snacks, beverages, and supplements during workouts are discussed, tailored to the specific demands of different exercise types.

Post-Exercise Nutrition and Recovery:

- The post-exercise period is critical for replenishing energy stores and facilitating muscle recovery.

- We explore the importance of post-exercise nutrition, including the timing and composition of meals and snacks to optimize recovery.

Tailoring Nutrition to Fitness Goals:

•	Different fitness goals, such as weight loss, muscle gain, or endurance training, require specific nutritional considerations.

•	Readers learn how to tailor their nutrition plans to align with their individual fitness objectives, ensuring optimal support for their training regimen.

Protein and Exercise:

•	Protein plays a key role in muscle repair and growth, making it essential for individuals engaged in regular exercise.

•	The chapter provides insights into protein requirements, sources, and timing to maximize its benefits for muscle health.

Carbohydrates for Endurance and High-Intensity Exercise:

•	Carbohydrates are a primary source of energy for endurance and high-intensity exercise.

•	Practical recommendations for carbohydrate intake before, during, and after such activities are discussed to sustain energy levels and promote recovery.

Fats and Exercise Performance: - While fats contribute to overall energy needs, their role in exercise performance varies based on the intensity and duration of the activity. - We explore how to incorporate healthy fats into the diet to support exercise goals.

Nutrient Timing for Enhanced Performance: - Nutrient timing involves strategically planning meals and snacks around exercise sessions to optimize performance and recovery. - The chapter offers guidance on nutrient timing and how to adjust nutritional intake based on workout schedules.

Supplements for Exercise: - Some individuals may choose to use supplements to enhance their exercise performance. - We discuss common supplements, their potential benefits, and considerations for their use, emphasizing the importance of obtaining nutrients primarily from whole foods.

Combining Strength Training and Nutrition: - Strength training has specific nutritional requirements to support muscle building and recovery. - Practical tips for aligning nutrition with strength training goals, including the importance of protein and calorie intake, are discussed.

Cardiovascular Exercise and Nutrition: - Cardiovascular exercise places unique demands on the body, necessitating specific nutritional strategies. - Readers learn how to tailor their nutrition plans for cardiovascular activities, including considerations for endurance and interval training.

Flexibility and Mind-Body Exercise: - Flexibility exercises and mind-body practices, such as yoga, have distinct nutritional considerations. - We explore how nutrition can support these activities, focusing on hydration, balanced meals, and mindful eating.

By the end of Chapter 11, readers will have gained a comprehensive understanding of the symbiotic relationship between exercise and nutrition. Armed with practical insights and strategies, they can optimize their nutritional choices to complement their fitness goals, enhance performance, and promote overall well-being.

Chapter Twelve

OVERCOMING CHALLENGES AND STAYING ON TRACK

Embarking on a journey towards a healthier lifestyle often comes with its fair share of challenges. Chapter 12 addresses common obstacles and provides practical strategies to help readers overcome setbacks, stay motivated, and maintain long-term commitment to their health and wellness goals.

 Identifying Common Challenges:

•   Acknowledging the existence of challenges is the first step in overcoming them. This section explores common obstacles individuals may face on their health and wellness journey, such as time constraints, emotional eating, and lifestyle disruptions.

Time Management and Prioritization:

•   Lack of time is a pervasive challenge. The chapter discusses effective time management strategies, emphasizing the importance of prioritizing health and wellness within busy schedules.

•   Practical tips for incorporating quick and efficient workouts, planning meals in advance, and making time for self-care are explored.

Emotional Eating and Stress Management:

•   Emotional eating can derail progress. Strategies for managing stress and emotional triggers are discussed, including mindfulness techniques, journaling, and seeking support.

• Readers learn to differentiate between physical hunger and emotional cues, cultivating a healthier relationship with food.

Plateaus and Adjusting Goals:

• Plateaus are a natural part of any journey. The chapter provides guidance on overcoming plateaus by adjusting goals, reassessing strategies, and introducing variety to workout routines and meal plans.

• Practical tips for staying motivated during periods of slower progress are included.

Social Pressures and Peer Influence:

• Social pressures and peer influence can impact lifestyle choices. Readers gain insights into navigating social situations, handling peer pressure gracefully, and seeking support from friends and family.

• Strategies for communicating health goals effectively and fostering a supportive social network are discussed.

Managing Setbacks and Building Resilience:

• Setbacks are inevitable, but building resilience is key to long-term success. The chapter explores how to bounce back from setbacks, learn from challenges, and cultivate a positive mindset.

•   Readers are encouraged to view setbacks as learning opportunities rather than reasons to abandon their goals.

Balancing Flexibility and Consistency:

•   Balancing flexibility with consistency is essential for sustainable habits. We discuss the importance of finding a middle ground, allowing for occasional indulgences while maintaining a commitment to long-term health.

•   Practical strategies for navigating special occasions, holidays, and unexpected events are provided.

Staying Motivated:

•   Sustaining motivation is an ongoing process. The chapter explores various techniques for staying motivated, including setting meaningful goals, tracking progress, and celebrating achievements.

•   Readers are encouraged to revisit their motivations regularly, adjusting goals and strategies as needed.

Building a Support System:

• A strong support system enhances the likelihood of success. Strategies for building a support network, including enlisting workout buddies, joining fitness communities, and seeking professional guidance, are discussed.

• The chapter emphasizes the importance of accountability and surrounding oneself with positive influences.

Celebrating Non-Scale Victories: - Celebrating victories beyond the scale is crucial for motivation. We explore non-scale victories, such as improved energy levels, enhanced mood, and increased confidence. - Readers are encouraged to recognize and celebrate the positive changes that extend beyond numerical measurements.

Creating a Sustainable Lifestyle: - Sustainable lifestyle changes are key to long-term success. The chapter provides guidance on transitioning from short-term habits to sustainable, lifelong practices. - Readers learn how to integrate health and wellness into their daily lives in a way that aligns with their values and priorities.

Seeking Professional Guidance: - In certain situations, seeking professional guidance can be beneficial. The chapter discusses the role of healthcare professionals, nutritionists, and fitness trainers in providing personalized support and guidance. - Readers are encouraged to consult with professionals to address specific health concerns or obtain expert advice.

By the end of Chapter 12, readers will have acquired valuable strategies for overcoming challenges, staying motivated, and maintaining a resilient and positive mindset on their health and wellness journey. Armed with practical insights, they can navigate setbacks and build sustainable habits for a healthier, more fulfilling lifestyle.

Chapter Thirteen

SUSTAINABLE WEIGHT MANAGEMENT

Sustainable weight management involves adopting long-term lifestyle changes that support a healthy body weight while prioritizing overall well-being. Chapter 13 explores the principles of sustainable weight management, providing readers with practical strategies for achieving and maintaining their desired weight in a balanced and healthful way.

Understanding Sustainable Weight Management:

• Sustainable weight management goes beyond short-term diets and quick fixes. The chapter introduces the concept of adopting lifestyle changes that are realistic, enjoyable, and maintainable.

• Readers learn to shift their focus from rapid weight loss to long-term health and wellness.

Setting Realistic Weight Goals:

• Setting realistic and achievable weight goals is a crucial first step. The chapter discusses how to establish personalized goals based on individual health needs, lifestyle, and preferences.

• Practical tips for breaking larger goals into smaller, manageable steps are provided.

The Role of Nutrition in Sustainable Weight Management:

• Nutrition is a cornerstone of weight management. We explore the principles of a balanced and sustainable diet, emphasizing whole foods, portion control, and mindful eating.

•   Readers learn how to make nutritional choices that support their weight goals while ensuring adequate nutrient intake.

Balancing Macronutrients for Satiety:

•   Balancing macronutrients, including carbohydrates, proteins, and fats, is essential for promoting satiety and preventing overeating.

•   Practical guidance on creating balanced meals that support feelings of fullness and satisfaction is discussed.

Physical Activity for Weight Maintenance:

•   Regular physical activity plays a vital role in weight management. The chapter explores different types of exercises, the importance of incorporating both cardio and strength training, and finding enjoyable activities for long-term adherence.

Building a Sustainable Exercise Routine:

•   Creating a sustainable exercise routine involves finding activities that align with individual preferences and lifestyle.

• Readers learn to set realistic fitness goals, gradually increase activity levels, and integrate movement into their daily lives.

Sleep and Stress Management:

• Sleep and stress directly impact weight management. The chapter discusses the importance of adequate sleep and effective stress management techniques.

• Readers gain insights into how sleep and stress affect weight and learn strategies for improving both.

Behavioral Strategies for Sustainable Change:

• Sustainable weight management requires addressing behavioral patterns. We explore techniques for identifying and modifying unhealthy habits, incorporating positive behaviors, and building a supportive environment.

• Practical tips for overcoming emotional eating, managing triggers, and developing mindful eating habits are discussed.

Creating a Supportive Environment:

• A supportive environment is crucial for sustainable weight management. The chapter provides guidance on fostering a healthy home and work environment, enlisting social support, and communicating weight management goals with loved ones.

Regular Monitoring and Adjustments: - Regular monitoring of progress allows for necessary adjustments. Readers learn how to track their weight, physical activity, and nutrition, making informed modifications to their plans as needed. - The chapter emphasizes the importance of flexibility and adaptability in the journey towards sustainable weight management.

Enjoying the Process and Celebrating Successes: - Enjoying the process is essential for long-term commitment. Readers are encouraged to find joy in their healthy lifestyle choices, celebrate successes, and cultivate a positive relationship with their bodies. - The chapter explores the role of mindset in sustainable weight management and encourages a shift towards self-compassion.

Seeking Professional Guidance: - In certain cases, seeking professional guidance can enhance the journey. The chapter discusses the role of healthcare professionals, dietitians, and fitness experts in providing personalized support and guidance. - Readers are encouraged to consult with professionals to address individual health needs and receive tailored advice.

By the end of Chapter 13, readers will have gained a comprehensive understanding of sustainable weight management principles and practical strategies for incorporating them into their lives. Armed with this knowledge, they can embark on a journey towards achieving and maintaining a healthy weight in a way that prioritizes long-term well-being and overall health.

Chapter Fourteen

MIND-BODY CONNECTION FOR HOLISTIC HEALTH

The mind-body connection is a powerful aspect of overall well-being, encompassing the interplay between mental, emotional, and physical health. Chapter 14 explores the significance of nurturing a positive mind-body connection, providing readers with insights and practical strategies to enhance holistic health.

Understanding the Mind-Body Connection:

• The mind-body connection acknowledges the intricate relationship between mental and physical health. The chapter introduces the concept, highlighting how thoughts, emotions, and attitudes can influence physical well-being.

• Readers gain insights into the interconnected nature of mental and physical health.

Stress and its Impact on Health:

• Stress is a common factor that can impact both mental and physical health. The chapter explores the physiological effects of stress, including the release of stress hormones and its implications on various bodily systems.

• Practical strategies for managing and reducing stress are discussed.

Mindfulness and Meditation:

• Mindfulness and meditation practices are powerful tools for enhancing the mind-body connection. We explore the benefits of these practices, including stress reduction, improved focus, and emotional regulation.

• Readers learn simple mindfulness and meditation techniques that can be incorporated into daily life.

Breathwork for Relaxation:

• Breathwork is a fundamental component of mind-body practices. The chapter delves into the importance of conscious breathing for relaxation, stress reduction, and promoting a sense of calm.

• Practical breathwork exercises and techniques are provided.

Positive Thinking and Affirmations:

• Positive thinking and affirmations contribute to a positive mindset. The chapter explores how cultivating positive thoughts and using affirmations can impact mental and emotional well-being.

• Readers learn to integrate positive thinking practices into their daily routines.

Gratitude and its Health Benefits:

• Practicing gratitude has been linked to various health benefits. The chapter discusses the positive impact of gratitude on mental health, emotional well-being, and overall life satisfaction.

• Strategies for incorporating gratitude practices into daily life are explored.

Emotional Intelligence:

• Emotional intelligence involves recognizing, understanding, and managing one's own emotions as well as empathizing with others. The chapter explores the importance of emotional intelligence in fostering a positive mind-body connection.

• Readers gain insights into developing emotional intelligence and building healthier relationships.

The Gut-Brain Axis:

• The gut-brain axis is a bidirectional communication system between the gut and the brain. The chapter explores the impact of gut health on mental well-being and the role of nutrition in supporting a healthy gut.

•   Practical tips for promoting gut health through dietary choices are discussed.

Movement and Mental Health:

•   Physical activity has profound effects on mental health. The chapter explores how exercise influences neurotransmitters, reduces stress, and improves mood.

•   Readers learn the mental health benefits of different types of physical activity and are encouraged to find enjoyable ways to stay active.

Sleep and Cognitive Function: - Adequate sleep is crucial for cognitive function and mental well-being. The chapter discusses the relationship between sleep and mental health, exploring strategies for improving sleep quality and establishing healthy sleep habits. - Readers gain insights into creating a conducive sleep environment and prioritizing restful sleep.

Holistic Nutrition for Mental Well-Being: - Nutrition plays a significant role in supporting mental well-being. The chapter discusses the impact of nutrient-dense foods on cognitive function, mood regulation, and overall mental health. - Practical tips for incorporating brain-boosting foods into the diet are provided.

Social Connections and Community: - Social connections contribute to emotional well-being. The chapter explores the importance of building and maintaining positive social relationships, fostering a sense of community, and seeking support when needed. - Strategies for nurturing social connections in both personal and community settings are discussed.

Art and Creativity for Emotional Expression: - Art and creativity provide outlets for emotional expression and self-discovery. The chapter explores how engaging in creative activities can positively impact mental and emotional health. - Readers learn about various forms of creative expression and how to incorporate them into their lives.

Seeking Professional Support: - In certain situations, seeking professional support is essential. The chapter discusses the role of mental health professionals, counselors, and therapists in providing guidance and support. - Readers are encouraged to prioritize their mental health and seek professional help when needed.

By the end of Chapter 14, readers will have gained a comprehensive understanding of the mind-body connection and practical strategies for enhancing holistic health. Armed with insights into mindfulness, stress management, positive thinking, and various other practices, they can foster a positive mind-body connection to support their overall well-being.

Chapter Fifteen

LONG-TERM WELLNESS AND FUTURE GOALS

In this chapter we shall be looking into the culmination of the knowledge and strategies presented throughout the diet book, focusing on the principles of long-term wellness and helping readers develop sustainable habits for a healthy and fulfilling life. It offers insights into maintaining progress, setting future goals, and embracing a holistic approach to well-being.

Reflecting on Progress:

• The chapter begins by encouraging readers to reflect on their journey thus far, celebrating achievements, and acknowledging personal growth.

• Reflection prompts guide individuals to recognize positive changes in habits, mindset, and overall well-being.

Embracing a Holistic Approach:

• Holistic wellness encompasses physical, mental, and emotional well-being. The chapter emphasizes the interconnected nature of these aspects and encourages readers to approach health holistically.

• Practical tips for integrating holistic practices into daily life are discussed.

Assessing Lifestyle Habits:

• Lifestyle habits play a crucial role in long-term wellness. The chapter guides readers in assessing their current habits, identifying those that contribute positively to well-being, and recognizing areas for improvement.

• Strategies for making gradual and sustainable changes are explored.

Establishing a Personalized Wellness Plan:

• Personalized wellness plans take into account individual preferences, goals, and lifestyle. Readers learn how to create a tailored plan that aligns with their unique needs and aspirations.

• The chapter provides guidance on setting realistic and meaningful goals for continued growth.

The Role of Mindful Eating in Long-Term Wellness:

• Mindful eating is highlighted as an essential practice for sustained well-being. The chapter revisits mindful eating principles, emphasizing its role in fostering a positive relationship with food and promoting overall health.

• Readers are encouraged to make mindful eating a foundational part of their long-term wellness journey.

Prioritizing Self-Care:

•	Self-care is fundamental to well-being. The chapter explores the importance of self-care practices, such as adequate sleep, stress management, and regular physical activity.

•	Practical self-care strategies that align with individual preferences are discussed.

Navigating Challenges with Resilience:

•	Challenges are inevitable, and resilience is key to overcoming them. The chapter revisits strategies for building resilience, emphasizing the importance of a positive mindset and adaptability.

•	Readers learn to view challenges as opportunities for growth and develop coping mechanisms.

Building a Supportive Environment:

•	A supportive environment plays a vital role in maintaining long-term wellness. The chapter discusses how to create and sustain an environment that encourages healthy habits, positive relationships, and personal growth.

•	Readers gain insights into fostering a support system that aligns with their wellness goals.

Integrating Physical Activity into Daily Life:

•	Regular physical activity is a cornerstone of long-term wellness. The chapter revisits the importance of staying active and provides tips for integrating enjoyable and sustainable forms of exercise into daily life.

•	Readers are encouraged to view physical activity as a lifelong commitment.

Continuing Education and Growth: - Lifelong learning contributes to personal growth and well-being. The chapter explores the benefits of continuing education, whether through books, courses, or new experiences. - Readers are encouraged to cultivate a curious mindset and embrace opportunities for ongoing learning.

Cultivating a Positive Mindset: - A positive mindset is a powerful asset for long-term wellness. The chapter revisits strategies for cultivating positivity, reframing challenges, and maintaining an optimistic outlook. - Practical exercises guide readers in fostering a positive mindset in various aspects of life.

Setting Future Wellness Goals: - Setting future goals is a crucial aspect of sustaining well-being. The chapter provides guidance on establishing realistic and meaningful goals, whether related to nutrition, fitness, personal development, or other aspects of life. - Readers learn to create a vision for their future wellness journey.

Celebrating Milestones and Non-Scale Victories: - Celebrating milestones and non-scale victories contributes to ongoing motivation. The chapter revisits the importance of acknowledging achievements, both big and small, and finding joy in the journey. - Readers are encouraged to regularly reflect on their progress and celebrate their successes.

A Lifetime of Health and Happiness: - The chapter concludes by reinforcing the idea that well-being is a lifelong journey. It encourages readers to view health and happiness as ongoing pursuits and to appreciate the continuous evolution of their wellness. - Practical tips for maintaining a positive and sustainable approach to long-term wellness are provided.

By the end of Chapter 15, readers will have gained valuable insights and practical strategies for sustaining long-term wellness. Armed with a holistic perspective, personalized wellness plans, and the tools to navigate challenges, individuals can embark on a lifelong journey towards health, happiness, and overall well-being.